A Doctor's Guide to Understanding & Managing

HIGH CHOLESTEROL

Dr Prabhat Das

MD, PhD, FACP

Better Health with Dr Das Series

Hardcover ISBN: 978-1-971672-18-2

Paperback ISBN: **978-1-971672-12-0**

eBook ISBN: **978-1-971672-13-7**

Printed in the United States of America

Disclaimer

This book is intended solely for educational and informational purposes. It is not meant to replace personal medical advice, diagnosis, or treatment.

Although I am a licensed physician, reading this book does not establish a doctor-patient relationship. Each individual's health condition, medical history, and risk factors are unique. Any medical decision should be made in partnership with your own healthcare professional who understands your specific situation.

Medical science is continually advancing. New research and updated guidelines may lead to changes in recommendations over time.

About the Author

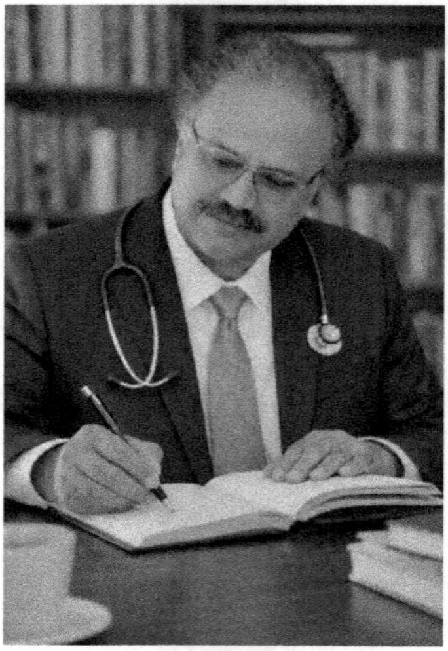

I am **Dr. Prabhat Das, MD, PhD, FACP**. My journey in medicine began in India, and for more than thirty five years I have had the privilege of practicing medicine in the United States. I am trained in **Internal Medicine, Pulmonary Diseases, and Critical Care**, and throughout these decades medicine has been far more than a career for me. It has been a lifelong calling rooted in learning, service, and deep respect for the people who place their trust in their physician.

Over the course of my medical career, I have cared for patients in many different settings. I have seen patients in my office for everyday health concerns, treated people in busy emergency rooms, managed complex illnesses in the hospital, and cared for the most critically ill patients in intensive care units. Thousands of patients have sat across from me during office visits. Many more have depended on careful decisions made during difficult and urgent moments in the hospital and ICU.

But medicine is not only about diagnoses, tests, and treatments. Every day I have listened to patients speak about their worries, their fears, their uncertainty, and often the many questions they hesitate to ask. Those conversations have taught me something profound. People want clear information, honest guidance, and reassurance they can trust. They want to understand their health so they can take better care of themselves and the people they love.

These experiences have shaped how I think about health, illness, prevention, and the deeply human side of healing.

Through the **"Better Health with Dr Das" series**, I hope to reach many individuals I may never meet personally in my office. Many people struggle quietly with health questions and confusing medical information. My goal in these books is simple. I want to explain important medical topics in a clear, practical, and reassuring way so that readers feel informed, confident, and empowered to make better decisions about their health. The information presented in these books is based on reliable scientific knowledge and decades of clinical experience.

If these books bring clarity to someone who feels confused, comfort to someone who feels worried, or practical help to someone trying to improve their health, then this effort will have been deeply worthwhile.

Helping people live healthier, better informed lives continues to be one of the greatest privileges and satisfactions of my professional life.

TABLE OF CONTENTS:

Introduction: Why Cholesterol Matters More Than Most People Think

Over the years, I have had this conversation with patients again and again. A patient comes into my office, sits down with a blood test report in hand, and says, "Doctor, my cholesterol is high. How worried should I be?"

It is a simple question, but behind it there is often a great deal of confusion.

Some people become anxious the moment they see an abnormal number. Others do not pay much attention because they feel perfectly fine. Many are caught in the middle. They know cholesterol is important, but they do not really understand what it is, why it matters, or what they should do next.

That uncertainty is very common, and it is exactly why I wrote this book.

Cholesterol is one of the most frequently discussed topics in medicine, yet it remains one of the most misunderstood. Almost everyone has heard the word. It appears in lab reports, doctor visits, advertisements, and everyday conversations. But for many people, it still feels vague, technical, and a little frightening.

Let me begin with a simple truth.

Cholesterol itself is not bad. In fact, your body needs it. Cholesterol is necessary for building cells, making certain hormones, producing vitamin D, and helping with digestion. Without it, the body could not function normally.

So the real problem is not cholesterol alone. The problem begins when cholesterol becomes too high, when the balance between different types of cholesterol becomes unhealthy, and when that imbalance quietly continues for years.

That is what makes cholesterol so important.

High cholesterol usually causes no symptoms. It does not make you feel sick. It does not usually cause pain. You may feel completely normal while, slowly and silently, changes are taking place inside your arteries. Over time, those changes can increase the risk of heart attack, stroke, and other serious problems.

But there is also very good news.

High cholesterol is one of the most manageable problems in modern medicine. With the right knowledge, sensible lifestyle changes, proper monitoring, and medication when needed, most people can improve their cholesterol and significantly reduce their risk.

This book was written to help you do exactly that.

I have written it in a simple, practical, and reassuring way. We will go step by step. You will learn what cholesterol really is, why it becomes high, how it affects the body, what the latest guidelines recommend, and what you can do to bring it under control. We will talk about food, exercise, weight, medications, side effects, newer injections, common myths, and real-life decisions that patients face every day.

My goal is not just to give you information. My goal is to give you **clarity, confidence, and a plan**.

I want this book to feel like a calm conversation with an experienced doctor, not a lecture filled with difficult medical language. I want you to finish this book feeling less worried, better informed, and more prepared to protect your health.

Because once you truly understand cholesterol, it stops feeling like a mysterious threat.

It becomes what it really is: a common medical problem that can be managed well with steady, informed, and practical steps.

Let us begin.

In the next chapter, we will start with the basics and make cholesterol simple, clear, and easy to understand.

Chapter 1: Cholesterol Made Simple

What It Is, Why You Need It, and Where Things Go Wrong

When patients first hear that their cholesterol is high, the reaction is often immediate.

They become concerned, sometimes anxious, and often assume that cholesterol is something harmful that should not be there at all.

But that is not quite true.

Let me start with a simple and reassuring statement:

Cholesterol is not your enemy. It is an essential part of your body.

The real issue is not cholesterol itself. The problem begins when its level becomes too high or when the balance between different types of cholesterol is disturbed over time.

Let us understand this clearly.

---

1. What Exactly Is Cholesterol?

Cholesterol is a soft, wax-like substance present in your blood and in every cell of your body.

It is not something foreign. Your body, especially your liver, produces most of the cholesterol it needs.

You also get some cholesterol from the food you eat, mainly from animal-based foods such as meat, eggs, and dairy products.

A simple way to think about cholesterol is this:

It is a **building material** your body uses every day.

Just as bricks are needed to build and maintain a house, cholesterol is needed to build and maintain your cells.

---

2. Why Your Body Needs Cholesterol

Many people are surprised to learn that cholesterol is actually useful.

It plays several important roles:

- It helps form the structure of your cell membranes
- It is used to produce important hormones
- It helps in making vitamin D
- It plays a role in digestion through bile formation

Without cholesterol, your body would not function properly.

So the goal is not to remove cholesterol, but to **maintain a healthy balance**.

---

3. How Cholesterol Travels in Your Blood

Cholesterol cannot travel freely in the blood. It needs carriers.

These carriers are called **lipoproteins**.

Understanding these carriers is important, because they determine whether cholesterol becomes helpful or harmful.

The two most important types are LDL and HDL.

---

4. LDL: The Cholesterol That Can Cause Problems

LDL stands for low-density lipoprotein.

It carries cholesterol from the liver to the rest of the body, which is necessary. But when LDL levels are high, excess cholesterol begins to deposit in the walls of arteries.

Over time, this can lead to narrowing of the arteries.

This is why LDL is commonly called "bad cholesterol."

In simple terms:

Too much LDL over time increases your risk of heart disease.

---

5. HDL: The Protective Cholesterol

HDL stands for high-density lipoprotein.

It works in the opposite way. It collects excess cholesterol from the bloodstream and carries it back to the liver, where it can be processed and removed.

Because of this protective role, HDL is called "good cholesterol."

Higher HDL levels are generally associated with lower cardiovascular risk.

---

6. Cholesterol and Your Diet: Clearing a Common Confusion

Many people believe that cholesterol comes only from food.

This is not correct.

Your body produces about 70 to 80 percent of your cholesterol. The rest comes from your diet.

This explains why:

- some people with healthy eating habits still have high cholesterol
- and some people with less healthy diets may not have very high levels

Diet matters, but it is only one part of the overall picture.

---

7. When Does Cholesterol Become a Problem?

Cholesterol becomes harmful when its balance is disturbed and remains so over time.

This usually means:

- LDL levels are too high
- HDL levels are too low
- this imbalance continues for years

When this happens, excess cholesterol begins to build up inside the walls of arteries.

This process is slow and silent, but over time it can increase the risk of heart attack and stroke.

---

8. A Simple Way to Think About It

At this stage, it is helpful to keep one clear idea in mind:

Cholesterol itself is not dangerous. Imbalance over time is.

Once you understand this, you move from fear to clarity.

And that is the first step toward effective management.

Chapter Summary

- Cholesterol is a natural and essential substance in the body
- It plays a key role in cell structure, hormones, and digestion
- LDL can become harmful when elevated

- HDL helps protect by removing excess cholesterol
- Most cholesterol is produced by the body itself
- Problems arise when cholesterol remains imbalanced over time

---

Action Plan

- Begin by understanding the basics of cholesterol
- Do not think of cholesterol as entirely "good" or "bad"
- Focus on balance rather than elimination
- Plan to check your cholesterol if you have not done so recently
- Start thinking in terms of long-term health

Looking Ahead

Now that you clearly understand what cholesterol is, an important question arises.

If high cholesterol can lead to serious problems, why do most people feel completely normal?

In the next chapter, we will explore why high cholesterol is often called a silent condition, and why waiting for symptoms can be risky.

Chapter 2: The Silent Threat

Why High Cholesterol Often Goes Unnoticed Until It Is Too Late

One of the most challenging aspects of high cholesterol is how quietly it behaves.

I still remember a patient who came to see me for a routine check-up. He felt well, remained active, and had no complaints. His blood test, however, told a different story. His cholesterol was significantly elevated.

When I explained this to him, he looked surprised and said, **"But doctor, I feel perfectly fine."**

That statement is very common. And it highlights the central problem with high cholesterol.

---

1. Why You Feel Normal Despite High Cholesterol

Most medical conditions give us warning signs.

Pain, fatigue, breathlessness, or discomfort alerts us that something is wrong.

High cholesterol does not behave that way.

It does not cause pain.
It does not affect your daily routine.
It does not make you feel sick.

That is because its effects are gradual and take place silently inside your blood vessels.

So you may feel completely healthy while changes are already beginning beneath the surface.

---

2. What Is Happening Inside Your Body

When LDL cholesterol remains elevated over time, it begins to deposit in the inner lining of your arteries.

At first, these deposits are very small and do not affect blood flow.

But your body reacts to these deposits. This leads to inflammation and the gradual formation of fatty streaks.

Over time, these changes develop into plaques that slowly narrow the arteries.

This process can continue quietly for many years.

---

3. Why the Body Does Not Warn You Early

The human body has an impressive ability to adapt.

Even as arteries begin to narrow, the body often maintains adequate blood flow, especially at rest.

Because of this, symptoms are delayed.

By the time symptoms appear, the condition may already be advanced.

---

4. When Symptoms Finally Appear

When symptoms do occur, they are often a sign that the disease has progressed.

Depending on the area affected, this may present as:

- chest discomfort during activity
- shortness of breath
- sudden blockage leading to a heart attack
- reduced blood flow to the brain causing a stroke

In many cases, these events are the first clear sign that cholesterol has been a problem for years.

---

5. The Importance of Early Detection

Because high cholesterol does not cause symptoms, **testing becomes essential**.

A simple blood test can identify abnormal cholesterol levels long before any damage becomes obvious.

This gives you a valuable opportunity.

You can act early, make changes, and reduce your risk before complications develop.

---

6. The Risk of Ignoring the Problem

It is natural to ignore what you cannot feel.

Many people delay testing or treatment because they feel well.

But the absence of symptoms does not mean the absence of disease.

Ignoring high cholesterol allows the process to continue silently, increasing the risk over time.

---

7. A Calm and Balanced Perspective

This chapter is not meant to create fear.

It is meant to create awareness.

High cholesterol is serious because it is silent. But it is also manageable because it develops slowly.

That gives you time.

Time to detect.
Time to act.
Time to prevent.

---

8. A Simple Real-Life Message

If there is one idea I want you to remember from this chapter, it is this:

Do not wait for symptoms to take action.

By the time symptoms appear, the disease has often been present for years.

Chapter Summary

- High cholesterol usually does not cause symptoms
- Damage develops slowly inside the arteries
- The body adapts, delaying warning signs
- Symptoms often appear late
- Serious events like heart attack or stroke may be the first sign
- Early detection through testing is essential

Action Plan

- Do not rely on how you feel to judge your health
- Get your cholesterol checked regularly
- Take abnormal results seriously
- Avoid delaying evaluation or treatment
- Focus on prevention

Looking Ahead

Now that you understand why high cholesterol remains hidden for so long, the next step is to understand your test results.

In the next chapter, we will break down your lipid report in a simple and practical way, so that you can clearly understand what your numbers mean.

Chapter 3: Understanding Your Numbers

LDL, HDL, Triglycerides, and What They Really Mean for You

At some point, almost every patient sits in front of me with a lab report and says,
"Doctor, I see all these numbers, but I don't really understand them."

That is completely understandable.

A lipid report can look technical and a little intimidating. But once you understand a few key ideas, these numbers become one of the most useful tools you have to protect your health.

Let us go through them step by step, in a simple and practical way.

---

1. The Lipid Panel: A Snapshot of Your Health

The standard test used to measure cholesterol is called a **lipid panel**.

It usually includes:

- Total cholesterol
- LDL (bad cholesterol)
- HDL (good cholesterol)
- Triglycerides

Sometimes, additional values such as non-HDL cholesterol or ApoB may be included.

Think of this test as a **snapshot**. It shows what is happening in your blood at a given time.

But to understand your risk, you need to look beyond a single number.

---

2. LDL: The Most Important Number

LDL, or low-density lipoprotein, is the main number we focus on.

It carries cholesterol from the liver to different parts of the body. When its level is high, excess cholesterol begins to deposit in the walls of arteries.

Over time, this contributes to plaque formation.

That is why LDL is called "bad cholesterol."

In practical terms:

- Higher LDL means higher risk
- Lower LDL means lower risk

For most people, improving LDL is the central goal of treatment.

---

3. HDL: The Protective Factor

HDL, or high-density lipoprotein, has a protective role.

It helps remove excess cholesterol from the bloodstream and returns it to the liver.

Because of this, it is called "good cholesterol."

In general:

- Higher HDL is beneficial
- Lower HDL may increase risk

However, it is important to remember that a high HDL level does not completely offset a high LDL level.

---

4. Triglycerides: The Metabolic Indicator

Triglycerides are another type of fat found in the blood.

They are closely related to how your body handles calories, especially excess sugar and refined carbohydrates.

High triglycerides are commonly seen in:

- obesity
- diabetes
- sedentary lifestyle
- diets high in processed foods

They are an important part of your overall risk profile.

---

5. Non-HDL Cholesterol: A Broader View

Non-HDL cholesterol includes all forms of cholesterol that can contribute to plaque formation.

It is calculated by subtracting HDL from total cholesterol.

This value gives a broader picture, especially in people with high triglycerides.

---

6. ApoB and Lp(a): When More Detail Is Needed

In some cases, additional tests can provide deeper insight.

ApoB (Apolipoprotein B) reflects the number of harmful cholesterol particles in the blood. It can be a more precise indicator of risk in certain individuals.

Lipoprotein(a), or Lp(a) is largely determined by genetics. Elevated levels can increase cardiovascular risk, even when other cholesterol values appear normal.

These tests are not needed for everyone, but they can be very helpful in selected situations.

---

7. What Is "Normal"? It Depends on You

This is a very important point.

There is no single "normal" value that applies to everyone.

Your ideal cholesterol levels depend on your overall risk.

For example:

- A lower LDL target is recommended for someone with diabetes or heart disease
- A slightly higher level may be acceptable in someone with low overall risk

This is why interpretation must always be personalized.

---

8. Trends Matter More Than One Number

It is easy to become concerned about a single test result.

But cholesterol management is not based on one report.

What matters more is the trend over time:

- Are your numbers improving?
- Are they stable?
- Are they gradually increasing?

Looking at patterns gives a much clearer picture than focusing on one value.

---

9. Making These Numbers Work for You

Once you understand your lipid report, it stops being confusing.

It becomes a guide.

A guide that helps you:

- understand your risk

- track your progress
- make informed decisions

That is a powerful shift.

Chapter Summary

- A lipid panel measures LDL, HDL, triglycerides, and total cholesterol
- LDL is the main focus for reducing risk
- HDL plays a protective role
- Triglycerides reflect metabolic health
- Non-HDL, ApoB, and Lp(a) provide additional insight
- Cholesterol values must be interpreted based on individual risk
- Trends over time are more important than a single result

Action Plan

- Obtain and keep a copy of your lipid reports
- Focus on understanding your LDL level first
- Pay attention to triglycerides and HDL
- Ask your doctor if additional tests are needed
- Track your results over time
- Discuss your numbers in the context of your overall health

Looking Ahead

Now that you understand your cholesterol numbers, the next question naturally arises.

Why do these numbers become abnormal in the first place?

In the next chapter, we will explore the causes of high cholesterol, including genetics, lifestyle, and several hidden factors that are often overlooked.

Chapter 4: What Causes High Cholesterol?

Genes, Lifestyle, and the Hidden Factors You Should Know

After reviewing their cholesterol report, many patients ask me a very direct question:

“Doctor, why is my cholesterol high?”

It is a simple question, but the answer is rarely simple.

In most cases, high cholesterol is not caused by just one factor. It is usually the result of several influences working together over time. Understanding these factors helps you approach treatment in a calm, balanced, and practical way.

Let us go through them clearly.

---

1. Genetics: The Influence You Inherit

One of the most important factors is your genetic background.

Some people naturally produce more cholesterol in the liver. Even with a healthy lifestyle, their levels may remain elevated.

A well-known example is **familial hypercholesterolemia**, an inherited condition in which cholesterol levels are high from a young age.

You should think about genetics if:

- your cholesterol is high at a younger age
- there is a family history of heart disease
- close relatives also have high cholesterol

In such cases, lifestyle alone may not be enough, and earlier treatment may be needed.

---

2. Diet: Important, but Not the Whole Story

Diet does play an important role, but it is often overemphasized as the only cause.

Foods that can raise cholesterol when consumed frequently include:

- saturated fats (red meat, butter, full-fat dairy)
- trans fats (processed and fried foods)
- diets high in refined carbohydrates and excess calories

At the same time, diets low in fiber and fresh foods can worsen cholesterol levels.

However, two people eating similar diets may still have very different cholesterol levels. This is because the body's response varies from person to person.

---

3. Lifestyle: Daily Habits That Add Up

Your daily habits have a strong influence on your cholesterol.

Factors that contribute to higher levels include:

- lack of physical activity
- excess body weight
- smoking
- excess alcohol intake

These habits often work together and gradually affect your metabolism.

Over time, they can increase LDL, lower HDL, and raise triglycerides.

---

4. Weight and Metabolic Health

Excess weight, especially around the abdomen, is closely linked to abnormal cholesterol levels.

It is often associated with:

- higher triglycerides
- lower HDL
- increased LDL in some individuals

Weight gain reflects changes in how your body processes fats and sugars.

Even modest weight loss can improve these patterns.

---

5. Age and Hormonal Changes

As we grow older, cholesterol levels tend to rise.

This is partly due to changes in metabolism and body composition.

In women, cholesterol levels often increase after menopause due to hormonal changes.

This makes regular monitoring more important with advancing age.

---

6. Medical Conditions That Affect Cholesterol

Certain health conditions can contribute to high cholesterol.

These include:

- diabetes
- hypothyroidism
- kidney disease
- liver conditions

In such cases, managing the underlying condition is an important part of cholesterol control.

---

7. Medications That Can Raise Cholesterol

This is often overlooked.

Some medications can affect cholesterol levels, including:

- certain steroids
- some blood pressure medications
- hormonal treatments

If cholesterol changes unexpectedly, it is worth reviewing medications with your doctor.

---

8. Hidden Contributors: Stress and Sleep

Less obvious factors also play a role.

Chronic stress and poor sleep can:

- affect hormones
- influence eating habits
- worsen metabolic balance

Over time, these factors can contribute to higher cholesterol.

---

9. A Balanced Way to Look at It

It is important not to blame yourself or focus on a single cause.

High cholesterol is usually the result of multiple factors.

The goal is not to find one reason, but to understand your overall situation and address what you can.

Chapter Summary

- High cholesterol is usually caused by multiple factors
- Genetics plays a major role in many individuals

- Diet and lifestyle significantly influence cholesterol levels
- Weight and metabolic health are important contributors
- Age and hormonal changes affect cholesterol over time
- Medical conditions and medications can raise cholesterol
- Stress and poor sleep also play a role

Action Plan

- Review your family history and personal risk factors
- Improve diet and lifestyle gradually
- Maintain a healthy level of physical activity
- Evaluate for underlying medical conditions if needed
- Review medications with your doctor
- Take a balanced and long-term approach

Looking Ahead

Now that you understand what causes high cholesterol, the next step is to understand what it actually does inside your body.

How does it lead to heart attack and stroke?

In the next chapter, we will explore this process in a simple and clear way, so that you can fully understand why managing cholesterol is so important.

Chapter 5: How Cholesterol Damages the Body

From Silent Build-Up to Heart Attack and Stroke

Patients often ask me a very honest question:
"Doctor, if my cholesterol is high, what is actually happening inside my body?"

That question matters.

Because once you clearly understand what cholesterol does inside your arteries, the importance of managing it becomes very real. It is no longer just about numbers on a report. It is about what is quietly happening over time.

Let us walk through this process step by step.

---

1. Your Arteries: Smooth and Healthy at the Start

Your arteries are the blood vessels that carry oxygen-rich blood from your heart to the rest of your body.

In a healthy state, the inner lining of these arteries is smooth, flexible, and clean. Blood flows freely without any resistance.

You can think of them as open, well-maintained pipes.

---

2. The First Change: Cholesterol Begins to Settle

When LDL cholesterol remains elevated over time, some of it begins to settle in the inner lining of the arteries.

At first, these deposits are tiny. They do not affect blood flow and do not cause any symptoms.

But the body recognizes these deposits as abnormal.

This triggers a response. Immune cells gather, and a mild inflammatory process begins.

This early stage is subtle and silent.

---

3. Plaque Formation: A Slow Build-Up

Over time, these early deposits grow into larger structures called **plaques**.

A plaque is not just cholesterol. It is a mixture of:

- cholesterol
- inflammatory cells
- calcium
- fibrous tissue

As plaques develop, they gradually thicken the artery wall.

This process is slow and can continue for many years without causing noticeable symptoms.

---

4. Narrowing of the Arteries

As plaques enlarge, they reduce the space inside the artery.

This means less room for blood to flow.

At first, the body compensates. You may not notice anything at rest.

But when your body needs more blood, such as during physical activity, the reduced flow may begin to matter.

In some people, this may lead to:

- chest discomfort during exertion
- reduced exercise capacity
- leg discomfort while walking

In others, there may still be no symptoms at all.

---

5. The Critical Moment: Plaque Rupture

The most dangerous event occurs when a plaque becomes unstable.

Sometimes, the surface of the plaque can rupture.

When this happens, the body tries to "repair" it by forming a blood clot.

This clot can suddenly block the artery.

If this occurs:

- in a heart artery, it leads to a **heart attack**
- in a brain artery, it leads to a **stroke**

These events often happen suddenly, without much warning.

---

6. Why This Process Matters

One of the most important things to understand is this:

This entire process develops slowly over many years.

That gives you an opportunity.

If you manage your cholesterol early, you can slow down or prevent this process. You can reduce plaque formation and lower your risk of serious events.

That is the power of prevention.

---

7. A Calm and Practical Perspective

It is easy to feel concerned when you hear about plaque and blockage.

But remember, this is not something that happens overnight.

You have time to act.

By controlling cholesterol, improving your lifestyle, and following appropriate treatment, you are directly influencing what is happening inside your arteries.

---

8. A Simple Way to Remember

If you remember one idea from this chapter, let it be this:

High cholesterol does not harm you suddenly. It harms you slowly, and that gives you time to prevent it.

Chapter Summary

- Arteries carry oxygen-rich blood throughout the body
- High LDL leads to cholesterol deposits in artery walls
- These deposits develop into plaques over time
- Plaques narrow arteries and reduce blood flow
- Plaque rupture can cause heart attack or stroke
- The process is slow and often silent

Action Plan

- Understand that cholesterol affects your arteries over time
- Take early steps to control cholesterol levels
- Focus on prevention rather than waiting for symptoms
- Maintain a consistent healthy lifestyle
- Follow medical advice to reduce long-term risk

Looking Ahead

Now that you understand how cholesterol damages the body, the next step is to understand your personal risk.

Not everyone with high cholesterol has the same level of risk.

In the next chapter, we will explore who is at risk, how to assess that risk, and how it guides treatment decisions.

Chapter 6: Who Is at Risk?

Understanding Your Personal Risk and Why It Matters

By now, you understand what cholesterol is and how it can affect your arteries.

But an important question remains:

"If two people have the same cholesterol level, will their risk be the same?"

In real life, the answer is often no.

This is one of the most important ideas in modern medicine. We do not treat cholesterol numbers alone. We treat **the person as a whole**.

Understanding your personal risk helps guide decisions about lifestyle, medications, and long-term care.

---

1. Risk Is More Than a Single Number

In the past, cholesterol levels were often considered in isolation.

Today, we take a broader view.

Your overall cardiovascular risk depends on a combination of factors, including:

- age

- blood pressure
- blood sugar levels
- smoking
- family history
- lifestyle habits

Looking at these together gives a much clearer picture.

---

2. Age: The Strongest Predictor

Age is one of the most powerful risk factors.

As the years pass, the effects of cholesterol gradually accumulate in the arteries.

Even if your cholesterol levels remain stable, your risk increases with time.

This is why regular monitoring becomes more important as you grow older.

---

3. Men and Women: Different Patterns of Risk

Men and women do not have identical risk patterns.

- Men tend to develop heart disease earlier
- Women usually have lower risk before menopause
- After menopause, women's risk increases

This change is related to hormonal shifts.

It is important not to underestimate cardiovascular risk in women, especially later in life.

---

4. Family History: The Hidden Clue

Family history provides important insight.

If close relatives have had:

- heart disease at a young age
- stroke
- very high cholesterol

your own risk may be higher.

This does not mean that problems are inevitable. But it does mean that early attention and prevention are especially important.

---

5. Medical Conditions That Increase Risk

Certain medical conditions significantly increase cardiovascular risk, even if cholesterol levels are not extremely high.

These include:

- diabetes
- high blood pressure
- chronic kidney disease

In these situations, cholesterol management becomes more aggressive because the overall risk is higher.

---

6. Lifestyle Factors: The Part You Can Change

Some risk factors are beyond your control, but many are not.

Lifestyle factors include:

- smoking
- lack of physical activity
- unhealthy diet
- excess body weight

The encouraging part is that these can be improved.

Changes in these areas can significantly reduce your overall risk.

---

7. Risk Calculators: Putting It All Together

Doctors often use **risk calculators** to estimate your likelihood of developing heart disease over the next 10 years.

These tools combine multiple factors and categorize risk into:

- low
- intermediate
- high

This helps guide treatment decisions, including whether medications are needed.

8. Risk Enhancers: The Extra Details

Sometimes risk is not clearly low or high.

In such cases, additional factors, called **risk enhancers**, are considered.

These include:

- family history of early heart disease
- elevated Lipoprotein(a)
- metabolic syndrome
- chronic inflammatory conditions

These details help refine decisions.

---

9. A Practical Perspective

Understanding your risk changes how you think about your health.

Instead of focusing only on numbers, you begin to see the bigger picture.

This allows for:

- more accurate decisions
- more appropriate treatment
- better long-term outcomes

Chapter Summary

- Cholesterol is only one part of cardiovascular risk
- Overall risk depends on multiple factors
- Age is a major contributor
- Men and women have different risk patterns
- Family history is important
- Medical conditions like diabetes increase risk
- Lifestyle factors significantly influence risk
- Risk calculators and enhancers help guide decisions

Action Plan

- Review your personal risk factors
- Do not focus on cholesterol numbers alone
- Ask your doctor about your overall risk level
- Address modifiable factors such as smoking and inactivity
- Take a proactive, long-term approach

Looking Ahead

Now that you understand your personal risk, the next step is to focus on detection.

When should you get tested? How often? Are there additional tests that can provide deeper insight?

In the next chapter, we will discuss testing, screening, and early detection in a clear and practical way.

Chapter 7: Tests, Screening, and Early Detection

When to Test, How Often, and What to Do with the Results

At this stage, many patients ask a very practical question:

"Doctor, how often should I check my cholesterol, and what do these tests really tell me?"

This is an important step.

Because cholesterol is a silent condition, **testing is your window into what is happening inside your body**. Without testing, you are simply guessing.

Let us make this simple and practical.

---

1. The Lipid Panel: Your Basic and Essential Test

The most important test for cholesterol is the **lipid panel**.

It measures:

- Total cholesterol
- LDL (bad cholesterol)
- HDL (good cholesterol)
- Triglycerides

This test forms the foundation of cholesterol evaluation.

It is simple, widely available, and highly useful.

---

2. When Should You Get Tested?

Most adults should have their cholesterol checked at least once in early adulthood.

After that:

- If your levels are normal and your risk is low, testing every few years is reasonable
- If you have risk factors such as diabetes, high blood pressure, or family history, testing should be done more often

After the age of 40, more regular testing becomes important.

The key idea is simple:

Do not wait for symptoms. Test proactively.

---

3. Fasting or Non-Fasting: What Should You Do?

Many people are unsure whether they need to fast before a cholesterol test.

In the past, fasting was always required.

Now:

- Many lipid tests can be done without fasting

- Fasting may still be useful when triglycerides need accurate measurement

If you are unsure, follow your doctor's advice.

But do not delay testing because of confusion about fasting.

---

4. Understanding Your Results in Context

When you receive your report, you may see labels such as "normal," "borderline," or "high."

These labels can be helpful, but they are not enough.

Your results should always be interpreted in the context of:

- your age
- your overall risk
- your medical history

For example, an LDL level that is acceptable for one person may be too high for someone with diabetes or heart disease.

---

5. Advanced Tests: When More Information Is Helpful

In some cases, additional tests can provide deeper insight.

Lipoprotein(a) or Lp(a)

- Largely determined by genetics

- Elevated levels increase cardiovascular risk
- Usually needs to be checked once in a lifetime

ApoB (Apolipoprotein B)

- Reflects the number of harmful cholesterol particles
- Can provide a more accurate assessment in certain situations

Coronary Calcium Score (CAC)

- A CT-based test that detects calcium in heart arteries
- Helps identify early plaque
- Useful when risk is uncertain

These tests are not needed for everyone, but they can be very helpful in selected cases.

---

6. How Often Should You Repeat Testing?

Cholesterol management is a long-term process.

Testing frequency depends on your situation:

- Stable and low-risk → less frequent testing
- On treatment or higher risk → more frequent monitoring

The goal is to track progress and make timely adjustments.

---

7. Avoiding Common Mistakes

Some common mistakes include:

- ignoring mildly abnormal results
- focusing too much on a single number
- delaying follow-up testing
- trying to interpret results without proper context

Avoiding these mistakes can make a significant difference.

---

8. A Practical Way to Think About Testing

Think of your cholesterol test as a **tool for guidance, not judgment**.

It helps you:

- understand your current status
- track your progress
- make informed decisions

Used correctly, it becomes one of your most valuable health tools.

Chapter Summary

- The lipid panel is the basic and essential test for cholesterol
- Testing should begin early and continue regularly
- Fasting is not always required
- Results must be interpreted in context
- Advanced tests like Lp(a), ApoB, and CAC can provide additional insight

- Regular follow-up testing is important

Action Plan

- Get a baseline lipid panel if you have not done so
- Repeat testing at appropriate intervals
- Do not rely only on "normal" or "high" labels
- Discuss your results with your doctor
- Ask about advanced testing if your risk is unclear
- Keep a record of your results over time

Looking Ahead

Now that you understand how and when to test your cholesterol, the next step is to understand how these results guide treatment.

What do current medical guidelines recommend? When should treatment begin? How low should cholesterol be?

In the next chapter, we will discuss the latest cholesterol guidelines in the United States in a clear and practical way.

Chapter 8: The Latest Cholesterol Guidelines in the USA

What Experts Recommend Today and What It Means for You

At this stage, many patients ask a very practical question:

"Doctor, based on all this, what do current guidelines actually recommend for me?"

This is where confusion often arises. Advice seems to change over time, and different sources may say different things.

Let me simplify this.

Guidelines are not meant to confuse you. They are meant to **bring clarity and consistency**. They are developed by expert groups after carefully reviewing years of scientific research.

Their goal is simple:

To reduce your risk of heart attack, stroke, and long-term complications.

---

1. Why Guidelines Keep Changing

Medicine is always evolving.

As new research becomes available, our understanding improves. What we believed ten years ago may be refined today.

In cholesterol care, research has clearly shown:

- long-term exposure to high LDL increases risk
- earlier control leads to better outcomes
- individual risk varies widely

Because of this, guidelines have moved toward a more **personalized and proactive approach**.

---

2. The Shift to a Risk-Based Approach

One of the most important changes in modern guidelines is this:

We no longer treat cholesterol numbers alone. We treat overall risk.

Your treatment plan depends on a combination of factors:

- age
- blood pressure
- diabetes
- smoking
- family history
- cholesterol levels

Based on these, patients are grouped into:

- low risk
- intermediate risk
- high risk
- very high risk

This helps doctors decide how aggressively to treat.

3. LDL: The Primary Target

Modern guidelines focus strongly on LDL cholesterol.

The key principle is:

Lower LDL leads to lower risk.

However, the target level depends on your risk category:

- Lower-risk individuals → moderate LDL targets
- Higher-risk individuals → lower LDL targets
- Very high-risk individuals → more aggressive lowering

There is no single number for everyone. The target is personalized.

---

4. When Should Treatment Begin?

Treatment decisions are based on both cholesterol levels and overall risk.

In general:

- Lifestyle changes are recommended for everyone
- Medications are considered when:
  - LDL is significantly elevated
  - overall risk is moderate or high
  - lifestyle measures are not sufficient

One important shift is that treatment is often started **earlier** in higher-risk individuals.

---

5. A Stepwise Approach to Treatment

Guidelines recommend a step-by-step approach:

1. Begin with lifestyle changes
2. Add a statin if needed
3. Add additional medications if targets are not reached

This allows treatment to be adjusted gradually and safely.

---

6. Risk Enhancers: Refining the Decision

Sometimes the risk is not clearly low or high.

In these situations, additional factors, called **risk enhancers**, are considered.

These include:

- family history of early heart disease
- elevated Lipoprotein(a)
- metabolic syndrome
- chronic inflammatory conditions

These help guide more precise decisions.

---

7. The Role of Additional Testing

Guidelines also emphasize the role of testing in refining risk.

Tests such as:

- Lipoprotein(a)
- ApoB
- coronary calcium score

can provide additional clarity, especially when treatment decisions are uncertain.

---

8. What This Means for You

For you as a patient, this approach is beneficial.

It means:

- your care is personalized
- your treatment is based on your actual risk
- decisions are made with greater accuracy

This leads to better prevention and better long-term outcomes.

---

9. A Simple Way to Remember

If you remember one idea from this chapter, let it be this:

Your treatment is not based on one number. It is based on your overall risk.

Chapter Summary

- Cholesterol guidelines are based on evolving scientific evidence
- Modern care uses a risk-based approach
- LDL is the primary treatment target
- Treatment is started earlier when appropriate
- Medications are added step by step
- Risk enhancers help refine decisions
- Additional testing can guide care

Action Plan

- Understand your overall risk, not just your cholesterol numbers
- Ask your doctor about your target LDL level
- Begin lifestyle changes early
- Do not delay treatment if recommended
- Stay informed about guideline-based care
- Participate actively in your health decisions

Looking Ahead

Now that you understand current guidelines, an important question follows.

How is this different from the way cholesterol was treated in the past?

In the next chapter, we will compare older and newer approaches in a simple and practical way, so you can clearly understand what has changed and why it matters.

Chapter 9: Old vs New Guidelines

What Has Changed, Why It Changed, and Why It Matters for You

At times, patients say to me,
"Doctor, a few years ago I was told something different. Why has the advice changed?"

It is a very reasonable question.

When medical advice evolves, it can feel confusing. But in reality, this change reflects progress. As we learn more, we refine our approach and improve patient care.

Cholesterol management has gone through such an evolution.

Let us look at this in a simple and practical way.

---

1. The Earlier Approach: Focus on Numbers

In the past, cholesterol care was largely centered around specific numbers.

The approach was straightforward:

- Keep LDL below a certain level
- Encourage general lifestyle changes
- Start medication when levels were clearly high

This method was helpful, but it had limitations.

It treated many patients in a similar way, without fully considering individual differences in risk.

---

2. The Modern Approach: Focus on Overall Risk

Today, the approach is broader and more personalized.

Instead of focusing only on cholesterol levels, we look at **the whole person**.

This includes:

- age
- blood pressure
- diabetes
- smoking
- family history
- lifestyle

Two patients with the same LDL level may have very different levels of risk.

That is why treatment is now tailored to the individual.

---

3. Earlier Intervention and Lower Targets

One of the most important changes is this:

We now act earlier and aim for lower LDL levels in higher-risk patients.

Research has shown that the longer your body is exposed to high LDL, the greater the risk of developing heart disease.

By lowering LDL earlier and maintaining lower levels over time, we can significantly reduce that risk.

---

4. More Treatment Options

In the past, treatment options were limited, mainly to statins.

Today, we have several additional therapies:

- ezetimibe
- PCSK9 inhibitors
- newer medications

These options help:

- achieve better cholesterol control
- provide alternatives for patients who cannot tolerate certain drugs

---

5. Personalized Care: The Biggest Change

Perhaps the most important shift is toward individualized care.

Modern guidelines recognize that:

- not everyone needs medication
- not everyone needs the same intensity of treatment
- decisions should reflect personal risk and preferences

This approach improves both effectiveness and patient comfort.

---

6. A Clear Comparison

Aspect	Earlier Approach	Current Approach
Focus	Cholesterol numbers	Overall cardiovascular risk
Treatment	Similar for most patients	Personalized approach
LDL Goals	Moderate targets	Lower targets for high-risk patients
Timing	Often delayed	Earlier intervention
Medications	Limited options	Multiple treatment options

---

7. What This Means for You

These changes are positive.

They mean:

- more accurate assessment of your risk
- more appropriate treatment decisions
- better long-term protection

If your treatment recommendations have changed over time, it is likely because newer evidence supports a better approach.

---

8. A Practical Way to Think About It

Instead of feeling uncertain about changing advice, think of it as refinement.

Medicine is becoming more precise, more personalized, and more effective.

And that benefits you.

Chapter Summary

- Earlier guidelines focused mainly on cholesterol numbers
- Modern guidelines focus on overall cardiovascular risk
- LDL targets are now lower for higher-risk individuals
- Treatment is started earlier when appropriate
- More medication options are available
- Care is now more personalized

Action Plan

- Stay updated with current medical advice
- Do not rely on outdated information
- Discuss your current plan with your doctor
- Focus on long-term prevention
- Be open to adjustments in your treatment

Looking Ahead

Now that you understand how cholesterol management has evolved, the next step is to focus on what you can do in your daily life.

Before medications, your most powerful tool is your lifestyle.

In the next chapter, we will explore how simple, consistent lifestyle changes can significantly improve your cholesterol and overall health.

Chapter 10. Lifestyle First: Your Most Powerful Treatment

Small Daily Changes That Make a Real Difference

After understanding cholesterol, risk, and guidelines, most patients turn to me and ask a very practical question:

"Doctor, what can I actually do in my daily life to improve this?"

This is the most important question in the entire journey.

Because before medications, before advanced treatments, before anything else, the foundation of cholesterol care is your **lifestyle**.

And the good news is this:

You have more control than you think.

---

1. Why Lifestyle Matters So Much

Cholesterol levels are not fixed. They respond to how you live each day.

Your habits influence:

- how your body produces cholesterol
- how it processes fats and sugars
- how your blood vessels respond over time

With the right changes, you can:

- lower LDL cholesterol
- increase HDL cholesterol
- reduce triglycerides
- improve overall heart health

These changes may not happen overnight, but they are steady and meaningful.

---

2. Consistency Is More Powerful Than Perfection

One of the most common mistakes I see is this:

Patients try to change everything at once.

They follow strict diets, intense exercise plans, and rigid routines. For a few weeks, they do very well. Then it becomes difficult to maintain.

They feel discouraged and stop.

A better approach is simpler:

Focus on consistency, not perfection.

- A daily walk is better than occasional intense workouts
- Balanced eating is better than short-term strict dieting
- Small changes done regularly are far more effective

Think long-term.

---

3. Weight: A Key Part of the Picture

Excess weight, especially around the abdomen, is closely linked to abnormal cholesterol.

It affects how your body handles fats, sugars, and insulin.

Even modest weight loss can make a meaningful difference:

- LDL may decrease
- triglycerides may improve
- overall metabolic health becomes better

You do not need rapid weight loss. You need steady progress.

---

4. Physical Activity: Simple and Effective

Regular movement is one of the most powerful tools you have.

Exercise helps:

- increase HDL (good cholesterol)
- reduce triglycerides
- improve circulation and overall fitness

You do not need complicated routines.

Simple options include:

- brisk walking
- cycling
- light strength exercises

Even 30 minutes on most days can make a noticeable difference.

---

5. Avoiding Harmful Habits

Some habits can undo much of your effort.

These include:

- smoking
- excessive alcohol intake
- prolonged inactivity

Smoking, in particular, damages blood vessels and lowers HDL.

Reducing or stopping these habits is one of the most important steps you can take.

---

6. Building a Routine That Works for You

Lifestyle change is not a temporary effort.

It is about building a routine that fits your life.

This means:

- setting realistic goals
- making gradual adjustments
- allowing flexibility

A routine that you can follow comfortably is far more valuable than a perfect plan that lasts only a short time.

---

7. A Long-Term Mindset

Cholesterol management is not a quick fix.

There will be times when progress feels slow. There may be setbacks.

That is normal.

What matters is that you continue.

Over time, your efforts add up in a meaningful way.

---

8. A Simple Thought to Remember

If you remember one idea from this chapter, let it be this:

Your daily habits matter more than occasional efforts.

Chapter Summary

- Lifestyle is the foundation of cholesterol management
- Daily habits influence cholesterol levels significantly
- Consistency is more important than perfection
- Weight management plays a key role
- Regular physical activity improves cholesterol

- Avoiding harmful habits is essential
- A long-term mindset leads to success

Action Plan

- Start with one or two small changes
- Build a consistent daily routine
- Include regular physical activity
- Work toward gradual weight improvement
- Avoid smoking and limit alcohol
- Focus on long-term habits, not short-term results

Looking Ahead

Lifestyle changes are powerful, and among them, diet plays a central role.

Many patients feel unsure about what to eat and what to avoid.

In the next chapter, we will take a closer look at diet and develop a clear, practical approach to eating for healthy cholesterol.

Chapter 11. Eating for Healthy Cholesterol

A Practical, Real-Life Way of Eating You Can Live With

Sooner or later, every patient asks me the same question: **"Doctor, what exactly should I eat?"**

It sounds simple, but it often becomes confusing.

There are too many diets, too many rules, and too many promises of quick results. Some plans are so strict that they work for a short time and then become impossible to maintain.

Let me simplify this for you.

You do not need a perfect diet. You need a sensible way of eating that you can follow comfortably for years.

That is what truly improves cholesterol and protects your heart.

---

1. Understanding Fats: Choosing the Right Kind

For many years, people were told to avoid all fats. We now know that this is not correct.

Some fats are helpful, while others can be harmful.

Healthier fats (unsaturated fats) can improve cholesterol balance:

- olive oil
- nuts such as almonds and walnuts
- seeds
- fatty fish

Fats to limit, especially when taken in excess:

- saturated fats found in red meat, butter, and full-fat dairy
- trans fats found in processed and fried foods

The goal is not to eliminate fat completely, but to **choose better fats and use them in moderation**.

---

2. Fiber: A Simple and Powerful Tool

Fiber plays an important role in lowering cholesterol.

It helps reduce LDL by limiting cholesterol absorption in the digestive system.

Good sources of fiber include:

- oats and whole grains
- fruits such as apples and berries
- vegetables
- beans and lentils

Increasing fiber intake is one of the easiest and most effective changes you can make.

---

3. Reducing Processed and Sugary Foods

Many modern diets include a large amount of processed food.

These foods are often:

- high in unhealthy fats
- high in sugar
- low in nutritional value

Examples include:

- fast food
- packaged snacks
- sugary drinks

Reducing these foods can significantly improve your cholesterol and overall health.

---

4. Portion Control: An Important but Overlooked Factor

Even healthy food can become a problem if eaten in large amounts.

Portion size matters.

You do not need to measure everything precisely, but it helps to be mindful.

Simple habits include:

- eating slowly
- avoiding unnecessary second servings
- paying attention to hunger and fullness

5. A Practical Eating Pattern

Instead of focusing on individual foods, it is more helpful to think about your overall pattern of eating.

A simple approach:

- include plenty of vegetables and fruits
- choose whole grains instead of refined grains
- use lean sources of protein
- include healthy fats in moderation

This approach is flexible and can be adapted to your preferences and culture.

6. Eating Outside and Real-Life Situations

Many patients do well at home but struggle when eating outside.

A few practical tips:

- choose grilled or baked options instead of fried
- avoid excessive sauces and processed foods
- control portion sizes
- balance your choices over the day

You do not need to avoid eating out. You need to make **better choices when you do**.

7. Avoiding Common Diet Mistakes

Some common mistakes include:

- following very strict diets that cannot be sustained
- eliminating entire food groups unnecessarily
- expecting rapid results

These approaches often lead to frustration.

A steady, balanced approach works better over time.

---

8. A Realistic Perspective

Your diet does not need to be perfect every day.

There will be occasions when you eat differently. That is normal.

What matters is your **overall pattern over weeks and months**, not a single meal.

---

9. A Simple Thought to Remember

If you remember one idea from this chapter, let it be this:

Eat better most of the time, not perfectly all the time.

Chapter Summary

- A balanced diet plays a major role in cholesterol management
- Not all fats are harmful; healthier fats can be beneficial
- Fiber helps reduce LDL cholesterol
- Processed and sugary foods should be limited
- Portion control is important
- A sustainable eating pattern is more effective than strict diets

---

Action Plan

- Replace unhealthy fats with healthier options
- Increase intake of fiber-rich foods
- Reduce processed and sugary foods
- Be mindful of portion sizes
- Make better choices when eating outside
- Focus on consistency rather than perfection

Looking Ahead

Diet is a key part of lifestyle, but it is not the only factor.

Physical activity, sleep, stress, and daily habits also influence your cholesterol.

In the next chapter, we will look beyond diet and explore these additional factors that play an important role in your overall health.

Chapter 12. Beyond Diet

Exercise, Weight, Sleep, Stress, and the Habits That Shape Your Health

By now, you have a good understanding of diet and its role in cholesterol.

But in my daily practice, I often see something interesting.

A patient will say,
"Doctor, I have improved my diet, but my cholesterol is still not where it should be."

That is when I explain an important point:

Diet is important, but it is only one part of the story.

Your body responds to a combination of habits. Physical activity, weight, sleep, stress, and daily routines all play a role in shaping your cholesterol and overall health.

Let us look at these factors in a practical and realistic way.

---

1. Physical Activity: A Powerful and Simple Tool

Regular movement is one of the most effective ways to improve cholesterol.

Exercise helps:

- increase HDL (good cholesterol)
- reduce triglycerides

- improve circulation and heart health

You do not need complicated routines or special equipment.

Simple activities such as:

- brisk walking
- cycling
- light strength exercises

done consistently can make a meaningful difference.

Even moderate activity for about 30 minutes most days of the week can help.

---

2. Weight: More Than Just a Number

Excess body weight, especially around the abdomen, is closely linked to abnormal cholesterol.

It reflects changes in how your body processes fats and sugars.

Weight gain is often associated with:

- higher triglycerides
- lower HDL
- increased cardiovascular risk

The encouraging part is that even modest weight loss can improve these patterns.

You do not need dramatic changes. Steady progress is enough.

---

3. Sleep: The Overlooked Factor

Sleep is often ignored when discussing cholesterol.

But poor sleep affects your body in important ways:

- it increases stress hormones
- it affects metabolism
- it can worsen cholesterol levels over time

Most adults need around 7 to 8 hours of good-quality sleep.

Improving sleep is a simple but effective step.

---

4. Stress: The Silent Influence

Stress is a part of life, but when it becomes chronic, it affects health.

It can lead to:

- unhealthy eating habits
- reduced physical activity
- hormonal changes

These effects can indirectly worsen cholesterol.

Managing stress does not require complex techniques.

Simple steps such as:

- regular activity
- relaxation time
- spending time with family

can help significantly.

---

5. Alcohol: Finding the Right Balance

Alcohol is often discussed with mixed messages.

Small amounts may have limited effects, but excessive intake can:

- increase triglycerides
- contribute to weight gain
- affect overall health

The safest approach is moderation, or avoiding alcohol if appropriate.

---

6. Smoking: A Major Risk Factor

Smoking has a clear and harmful effect on cholesterol and blood vessels.

It:

- lowers HDL
- damages artery walls
- increases cardiovascular risk

Stopping smoking is one of the most important decisions for your health.

---

7. Putting It All Together

When you look at these factors together, a clear message emerges.

Your daily routine shapes your long-term health.

It is not one single change, but a combination of small, consistent habits that make the difference.

---

8. A Simple Thought to Remember

If you remember one idea from this chapter, let it be this:

What you do every day matters more than what you do occasionally.

Chapter Summary

- Cholesterol is influenced by multiple lifestyle factors beyond diet
- Regular physical activity improves cholesterol
- Weight management plays a key role
- Good sleep supports metabolic health
- Stress can indirectly affect cholesterol
- Alcohol should be limited
- Smoking significantly increases risk

Action Plan

- Include regular physical activity in your routine
- Work toward a healthy body weight
- Aim for consistent, good-quality sleep
- Manage stress with simple daily habits
- Limit alcohol intake
- Stop smoking if applicable
- Build a sustainable daily routine

Looking Ahead

So far, we have focused on lifestyle, which forms the foundation of cholesterol management.

However, in many cases, lifestyle changes alone may not be enough.

In the next chapter, we will discuss cholesterol-lowering medications, when they are needed, how they work, and how they can be used safely and effectively.

Chapter 13. Cholesterol Medications Demystified

Statins and Other Medicines Explained in a Clear and Reassuring Way

At this point in the journey, many patients pause and ask me, **"Doctor, do I really need medication?"**

I can understand that hesitation.

No one likes the idea of starting a long-term medicine. There is often concern about side effects, dependency, or whether lifestyle changes alone might be enough.

Let me address this in a calm and practical way.

Cholesterol medications are not a failure. They are a tool. A tool that, when used appropriately, can significantly reduce your risk of heart attack and stroke.

---

1. When Do You Really Need Medication?

Not everyone with high cholesterol needs medication immediately.

In general, medicines are considered when:

- LDL remains elevated despite lifestyle changes
- overall cardiovascular risk is moderate to high
- there is a history of heart disease or stroke
- genetic conditions cause very high cholesterol

The decision is always individualized.

The goal is not simply to lower a number, but to **reduce your long-term risk**.

---

2. Statins: The Foundation of Treatment

Statins are the most commonly used and most studied cholesterol medications.

They work by reducing cholesterol production in the liver, which lowers LDL levels in the blood.

Common examples include:

- atorvastatin
- rosuvastatin
- simvastatin

Statins have been used for many years and have consistently shown:

- significant reduction in LDL cholesterol
- reduced risk of heart attack and stroke
- improved long-term outcomes

For most patients who need medication, statins are the first step.

---

3. Ezetimibe: A Useful Add-On

Ezetimibe works differently.

It reduces the absorption of cholesterol from the intestine.

It is often used:

- when statins alone are not enough
- when higher doses of statins are not well tolerated

It is generally well tolerated and works well in combination with statins.

---

4. Bempedoic Acid: Another Oral Option

Bempedoic acid is a newer oral medication.

It lowers cholesterol through a pathway different from statins.

It may be considered in:

- patients who cannot tolerate statins
- those needing additional LDL reduction

It provides another option for individualized treatment.

---

5. Combination Therapy: Working Together for Better Results

In many patients, one medication may not be enough.

Doctors often use combinations such as:

- statin plus ezetimibe

- statin plus other agents

This allows better cholesterol control while keeping individual drug doses safe.

---

6. How Long Will You Need Medication?

This is one of the most common concerns.

In most cases, cholesterol medications are taken long term.

This is because the underlying tendency for high cholesterol usually continues.

If medication is stopped without proper guidance, cholesterol levels often rise again.

It is helpful to think of medication as part of **ongoing protection**, not a temporary fix.

---

7. Addressing Common Concerns

Let me address a few common worries I hear from patients:

- "Will I become dependent on it?"
  No. The medication is not addictive. It is simply managing an ongoing condition.
- "Can I stop once my numbers improve?"
  Improvement often happens because of the medication. Stopping may reverse that progress.

- "Can lifestyle replace medication?"
  Sometimes yes, but not always. In many cases, both are needed together.

---

8. A Balanced Perspective

It is natural to feel cautious about medications.

But it is equally important to recognize their benefits.

When used appropriately, these medicines:

- are effective
- are generally safe
- significantly reduce long-term risk

---

9. A Simple Thought to Remember

If you remember one idea from this chapter, let it be this:

Medication is not the opposite of lifestyle. It works together with lifestyle.

Chapter Summary

- Medications are recommended based on cholesterol levels and overall risk
- Statins are the mainstay of treatment
- Ezetimibe and other drugs provide additional options

- Combination therapy may be needed in some cases
- Treatment is individualized
- Medications are usually required long term

Action Plan

- Discuss clearly with your doctor whether medication is needed
- Understand the purpose of each prescribed medicine
- Take medications regularly as advised
- Do not stop medication without medical guidance
- Combine medication with lifestyle changes
- Keep regular follow-up

Looking Ahead

While medications are effective, it is natural to have concerns about safety and side effects.

In the next chapter, we will discuss side effects in a clear and reassuring way, so that you know what to expect and how to handle it confidently.

Chapter 14: Medicines -Side Effects and Safety

What to Expect, What to Watch For, and How to Stay Confident with Treatment

Once medication enters the picture, a very natural concern follows.

Patients often ask me,
"Doctor, are these medicines safe?"

Sometimes this concern comes from personal experience. Sometimes from something heard from a friend, or read online. And sometimes it is simply the natural hesitation that comes with starting a long-term treatment.

Let us talk about this clearly and calmly.

Most cholesterol medications, especially statins, are well studied, widely used, and generally safe.

Like all medicines, they can have side effects. But serious problems are uncommon.

Understanding this properly helps replace fear with confidence.

---

1. What Most Patients Actually Experience

The first and most reassuring point is this:

Most patients do not experience significant side effects.

Many people take these medications for years without any noticeable problem.

Some patients may notice mild symptoms, especially when starting treatment, such as:

- mild muscle aches
- a sense of fatigue
- occasional digestive discomfort

In many cases, these symptoms improve over time or with small adjustments.

---

2. Muscle Symptoms: The Most Discussed Issue

Muscle-related symptoms are the most commonly talked about.

Patients may describe:

- soreness
- stiffness
- mild discomfort

In most cases:

- symptoms are mild
- they improve with dose adjustment
- or a change in medication

Severe muscle injury is very rare.

If symptoms are persistent, it is important to discuss them rather than ignore them.

3. Liver Effects: What You Should Know

Another common concern is the effect of statins on the liver.

Statins can cause mild changes in liver enzyme levels, but **serious liver problems are uncommon**.

Doctors may check blood tests after starting treatment to ensure everything remains safe.

For most patients, these medications are well tolerated by the liver.

---

4. Blood Sugar and Diabetes

There has been discussion about statins and blood sugar.

In some individuals, statins may slightly increase blood sugar levels.

However:

- the increase is usually small
- the benefit in reducing heart disease risk is much greater

For patients with diabetes or prediabetes, monitoring is important, but statins remain a valuable treatment.

5. What to Do If You Notice Symptoms

If you notice any symptoms after starting medication, the most important step is simple:

Do not stop the medication on your own.

Instead:

- note the symptoms clearly
- discuss them with your doctor
- review timing and possible causes

In many cases, the solution may be:

- adjusting the dose
- switching to a different medication
- or confirming that symptoms are not related to the drug

---

6. Avoiding Unnecessary Fear

In today's world, it is easy to come across alarming information.

Stories about side effects can sometimes be exaggerated or taken out of context.

It is important to rely on balanced, evidence-based information.

A calm and informed approach helps you make better decisions.

---

7. Balancing Benefit and Risk

Every treatment in medicine involves a balance.

In cholesterol management:

- the risk of side effects is generally low
- the benefit in preventing heart attack and stroke is significant

For most patients who need treatment, the benefits clearly outweigh the risks.

---

8. Staying Comfortable with Long-Term Treatment

It is important to feel comfortable with your treatment plan.

This comes from:

- understanding the purpose of the medication
- knowing what to expect
- having open communication with your doctor

Confidence grows when you are informed.

---

9. A Simple Thought to Remember

If you remember one idea from this chapter, let it be this:

Most patients tolerate these medications well, and the benefits are usually much greater than the risks.

Chapter Summary

- Cholesterol medications are generally safe and well tolerated
- Most patients experience no significant side effects
- Mild muscle symptoms are the most common issue
- Serious side effects are rare
- Regular monitoring ensures safety
- Benefits of treatment usually outweigh the risks

Action Plan

- Start medication with a clear understanding
- Be aware of possible mild side effects
- Report symptoms early
- Do not stop medication without medical advice
- Keep regular follow-up appointments
- Focus on long-term benefits

Looking Ahead

While traditional medications work well for most patients, newer treatments have expanded our options.

In the next chapter, we will explore advanced therapies, including injections and newer medicines, that are changing the way we manage cholesterol today.

Chapter 15: New and Advanced Treatments

Injections, New Therapies, and What They Mean for You

By now, you have a clear understanding of lifestyle changes and standard medications.

For most patients, these are enough.

But in real clinical practice, I often see patients who ask:

"Doctor, I am doing everything right, but my cholesterol is still high. What next?"

This is where newer and advanced treatments come in.

Over the past several years, cholesterol care has evolved significantly. We now have additional options that can help patients who need more support.

Let us understand these in a simple and practical way.

---

1. Why New Treatments Are Needed

Even with the best use of statins, some patients do not reach their target LDL levels.

This may happen because:

- their starting cholesterol is very high

- genetic factors are involved
- they cannot tolerate higher doses of statins

In such cases, additional therapies help us achieve better control.

---

2. PCSK9 Inhibitors: A Major Step Forward

One of the most important advances in recent years is the development of **PCSK9 inhibitors**.

These are injectable medications that help the liver remove more LDL cholesterol from the blood.

They can reduce LDL levels significantly, often more than what can be achieved with statins alone.

Common examples include:

- evolocumab
- alirocumab

These injections are usually given once every 2 to 4 weeks.

They are especially useful for:

- patients with very high cholesterol
- those with known heart disease
- individuals who do not reach targets with standard therapy

---

3. Inclisiran: A Convenient New Option

Inclisiran is another newer injectable treatment.

It works by reducing the production of a protein involved in cholesterol regulation.

Its main advantage is convenience.

It is given:

- initially
- then after a few months
- and then about twice a year

This can be helpful for patients who prefer fewer doses and a simpler schedule.

---

4. Bempedoic Acid: An Oral Alternative

For patients who prefer tablets or cannot tolerate statins, **bempedoic acid** is another option.

It works in the liver through a different mechanism and helps lower LDL cholesterol.

It can be used:

- alone
- or along with other medications

This adds flexibility in treatment planning.

---

5. Combination Therapy: A Practical Approach

In many patients, combining treatments provides the best results.

For example:

- statin plus ezetimibe
- statin plus newer agents

This approach allows:

- better cholesterol control
- lower doses of individual drugs
- improved tolerability

---

6. Who Should Consider These Treatments?

These advanced therapies are not needed for everyone.

They are generally considered for:

- patients at very high cardiovascular risk
- those who do not achieve target LDL levels
- individuals with genetic cholesterol disorders
- patients who cannot tolerate standard medications

The decision is always personalized.

---

7. Cost and Access

One practical issue with newer treatments is cost.

Injectable therapies can be expensive, and insurance coverage varies.

However, for selected patients, the benefits can be significant and justify their use.

---

8. Looking Toward the Future

Research in cholesterol treatment continues to progress.

New therapies aim to:

- improve effectiveness
- reduce side effects
- simplify treatment

This is encouraging, especially for patients who have struggled to control cholesterol in the past.

---

9. A Simple Thought to Remember

If you remember one idea from this chapter, let it be this:

If standard treatment is not enough, there are additional options available.

Chapter Summary

- New treatments are available for patients needing additional support
- PCSK9 inhibitors are effective injectable therapies
- Inclisiran offers a convenient dosing schedule
- Bempedoic acid provides an oral alternative
- Combination therapy is often used for better control
- These treatments are used selectively
- Cost and access are important considerations

Action Plan

- Discuss with your doctor whether advanced treatments are appropriate
- Understand the benefits and limitations of each option
- Consider cost and insurance coverage
- Follow your treatment plan consistently
- Continue lifestyle measures alongside medication

Looking Ahead

Cholesterol management is not the same for everyone.

Certain situations require a more individualized approach.

In the next chapter, we will discuss special situations such as diabetes, aging, and inherited conditions, where treatment decisions need to be tailored more carefully.

Chapter 16. Special Situations

Diabetes, Aging, Family History, and When Care Needs to Be Personalized

Up to this point, we have discussed cholesterol in a general way.

But in real life, no two patients are exactly the same.

Each person brings a unique combination of age, medical conditions, family history, and lifestyle. Because of this, cholesterol management often needs to be adjusted thoughtfully.

In this chapter, we will look at some common situations where a more personalized approach becomes especially important.

---

1. Cholesterol in Diabetes: Higher Risk, Earlier Action

If there is one condition that significantly increases cardiovascular risk, it is diabetes.

Even when cholesterol levels are only moderately elevated, the presence of diabetes increases the likelihood of heart disease.

This happens because diabetes affects blood vessels and accelerates plaque formation.

For this reason:

- treatment is often started earlier
- LDL targets are usually lower
- medications are commonly recommended

In patients with diabetes, cholesterol control is a key part of overall care.

---

2. Cholesterol in Older Adults: A Balanced Approach

As we age, cholesterol levels tend to rise and cardiovascular risk increases.

However, treatment in older adults requires balance.

We must consider:

- overall health and functional status
- presence of other medical conditions
- tolerance to medications
- personal preferences

Some older adults benefit greatly from treatment, while others may require a more cautious approach.

The goal is always to improve quality of life while reducing meaningful risk.

---

3. Familial Hypercholesterolemia: The Genetic Factor

Some individuals have high cholesterol primarily due to inherited causes.

Familial hypercholesterolemia is an important example.

These patients often:

- have very high cholesterol from a young age
- have a strong family history
- develop heart disease earlier

In such cases:

- early diagnosis is critical
- treatment is usually more aggressive
- family members should also be screened

---

4. Family Screening: Protecting More Than One Person

If high cholesterol is found to have a genetic component, it is important to think beyond one individual.

Close relatives may also be affected.

Screening family members can:

- identify problems early
- allow early treatment
- prevent future complications

This is a simple but powerful step.

---

5. Women and Cholesterol: Important Considerations

Cholesterol patterns differ between men and women.

- Women generally have lower risk before menopause
- After menopause, cholesterol levels tend to rise
- Cardiovascular risk increases with age

Additional considerations include:

- pregnancy-related changes
- use of hormonal therapies

It is important not to underestimate cardiovascular risk in women, especially later in life.

---

6. When Standard Medications Are Not Tolerated

Some patients find it difficult to tolerate certain medications.

They may experience side effects or feel uncomfortable continuing treatment.

In such cases:

- lower doses may be tried
- alternative medications may be used
- combination therapy may be considered

The goal is always to find a plan that is both effective and acceptable.

7. Multiple Conditions: The Whole-Patient Approach

Many patients have more than one health condition.

Conditions such as:

- high blood pressure
- kidney disease
- obesity

can interact with cholesterol and increase overall risk.

Treatment should always address the whole person, not just one number.

---

8. A Personalized Perspective

The most important message of this chapter is simple:

Cholesterol management must be individualized.

There is no one plan that fits everyone.

Your care should reflect your specific situation, your risk, and your preferences.

---

9. A Simple Thought to Remember

If you remember one idea from this chapter, let it be this:

Your treatment should be tailored to you, not based on a general rule.

Chapter Summary

- Cholesterol management must be individualized
- Diabetes significantly increases cardiovascular risk
- Treatment in older adults requires balance
- Genetic conditions require early and often aggressive care
- Family screening is important
- Women have unique risk patterns
- Alternative approaches are available when needed
- Multiple conditions should be managed together

Action Plan

- Discuss your individual situation with your doctor
- Inform your doctor about all medical conditions
- Consider family screening if needed
- Follow a personalized treatment plan
- Stay consistent with monitoring
- Be open to adjustments over time

Looking Ahead

You now have a strong understanding of cholesterol, its causes, risks, and treatments.

The next step is to bring everything together into a simple and practical plan.

In the next chapter, we will create a clear step-by-step plan of action that you can follow to take control of your cholesterol and your long-term health.

Chapter 17: Your Personal Plan of Action

A Clear, Practical Path to Taking Control of Your Cholesterol

You have now reached an important point in this journey.

You understand cholesterol, your risk, lifestyle changes, medications, and even advanced treatments. But knowledge alone is not enough.

What truly matters is this:

What will you do starting today?

Patients often ask me,
"Doctor, can you give me a simple plan?"

That is exactly what this chapter is about.

---

1. Know Where You Stand

Every plan begins with clarity.

Before you make changes, take a moment to understand:

- your latest cholesterol numbers
- your overall cardiovascular risk
- any associated conditions such as diabetes or high blood pressure

This becomes your starting point.

Without this, it is difficult to measure progress.

---

2. Set Clear and Realistic Goals

Your goals should be practical and personalized.

These may include:

- reaching a target LDL level
- improving your daily activity
- reducing excess weight
- building better eating habits

Avoid setting unrealistic targets.

Steady, achievable goals are more effective than ambitious plans that are hard to maintain.

---

3. Build a Simple Daily Routine

Health is shaped by daily habits.

A practical routine may include:

- regular physical activity, even a daily walk
- balanced meals with reasonable portions
- consistent sleep
- time for relaxation

The goal is not complexity. It is regularity.

---

4. Combine Lifestyle and Medication When Needed

Some patients feel they must choose between lifestyle changes and medication.

In reality, the best results often come from using both.

- Lifestyle improves overall health
- Medication helps achieve target levels more effectively

Together, they provide stronger protection.

---

5. Track Your Progress

Cholesterol management is gradual.

Tracking helps you see:

- whether your efforts are working
- how your body is responding
- when adjustments are needed

Keep a record of:

- lipid reports
- weight changes
- activity patterns

Even small improvements are meaningful.

---

6. Stay Connected with Your Doctor

This is not a one-time decision.

Regular follow-up allows:

- adjustment of treatment
- monitoring for side effects
- fine-tuning your plan

Think of this as an ongoing partnership.

---

7. Stay Consistent, Even When Progress Feels Slow

There will be times when progress seems slow.

You may feel that your efforts are not making a big difference.

That is normal.

Consistency over time is what produces real change.

---

8. Focus on Direction, Not Perfection

Life is not perfect.

There will be days when you miss exercise or eat differently.

That is part of being human.

What matters is the overall direction of your habits, not occasional setbacks.

---

9. A Simple Thought to Remember

If you remember one idea from this chapter, let it be this:

A clear plan, followed consistently, will always work better than a perfect plan followed occasionally.

Chapter Summary

- A clear plan is essential for effective cholesterol management
- Understanding your baseline helps guide action
- Goals should be realistic and personalized
- Daily habits form the foundation of success
- Lifestyle and medications often work best together
- Regular monitoring helps track progress
- Consistency is the key to long-term success

Action Plan

- Know your cholesterol levels and risk
- Set simple and achievable goals
- Build a consistent daily routine
- Combine lifestyle and medication when needed
- Track your progress regularly
- Maintain follow-up with your doctor
- Stay patient and consistent

Looking Ahead

Even with a clear plan, questions and doubts are natural.

In the next chapter, we will address frequently asked questions, helping you feel more confident and clear as you move forward.

Chapter 18. Frequently Asked Questions

Clear Answers to Real Questions Patients Often Ask

Even after understanding cholesterol, many patients still have practical questions.

In my daily practice, I hear the same concerns again and again. These are thoughtful questions, and addressing them clearly can make a big difference in how confident you feel about your health.

Let us go through some of the most common ones.

---

1. "If I Feel Fine, Do I Really Need Treatment?"

Yes, if your cholesterol is high or your risk is elevated.

High cholesterol usually does not cause symptoms. You may feel completely well while changes are slowly occurring inside your arteries.

Treatment is meant to **prevent future problems**, not to treat current symptoms.

---

2. "Can I Control Cholesterol Without Medication?"

In some cases, yes.

If your cholesterol is only mildly elevated and your overall risk is low, lifestyle changes may be enough.

However, if your risk is higher or cholesterol levels are significantly elevated, medication may be necessary.

The decision should be based on proper evaluation, not guesswork.

---

3. "Are Statins Safe for Long-Term Use?"

Yes.

Statins have been studied extensively and are widely used.

Most patients tolerate them well. Serious side effects are uncommon, and regular monitoring helps ensure safety.

---

4. "Can I Stop Medication Once My Numbers Improve?"

This is a common misunderstanding.

Cholesterol levels often improve because of treatment.

If medication is stopped, levels may rise again.

Most patients need long-term management, though adjustments can be made over time.

---

5. “Do Natural Remedies Work?”

Lifestyle changes such as diet and exercise are very effective.

However, many supplements marketed as “natural” have limited scientific evidence.

It is important not to rely only on unproven remedies, especially if your risk is significant.

---

6. “How Often Should I Check My Cholesterol?”

It depends on your situation.

- Low-risk and stable → every few years
- Higher risk or on treatment → more frequent testing

Your doctor can guide you.

---

7. “Does High Cholesterol Always Lead to Heart Disease?”

No.

It increases risk, but it does not guarantee disease.

Many factors influence outcomes, including lifestyle and genetics.

The goal is to reduce risk as much as possible.

---

8. "Is Diet Alone Enough?"

Diet is very important, but not always sufficient.

Some individuals need medication despite good dietary habits, especially if genetics play a role.

---

9. "What If I Miss a Dose of My Medication?"

This is a practical concern.

- If you miss a dose occasionally, take the next scheduled dose
- Do not double the dose unless advised
- Try to take medication at the same time daily

If missed doses happen frequently, discuss with your doctor.

---

10. "Can I Drink Alcohol While on Cholesterol Medication?"

In moderation, alcohol may be acceptable for some individuals.

However:

- excessive alcohol can raise triglycerides
- it may affect liver function

It is best to discuss your individual situation with your doctor.

11. “What Questions Should I Ask My Doctor?”

This is very important.

Consider asking:

- What is my overall risk?
- What should my target LDL be?
- Do I need medication now?
- Are there alternative options?
- How often should I follow up?

Good communication leads to better care.

---

12. A Simple Thought to Remember

If you remember one idea from this chapter, let it be this:

There are no “silly” questions when it comes to your health. Clarity is always better than confusion.

Chapter Summary

- High cholesterol often requires treatment even without symptoms
- Lifestyle changes may be sufficient in some cases
- Statins are generally safe for long-term use
- Cholesterol management is usually ongoing
- Natural remedies should be approached with caution

- Testing frequency depends on individual risk
- Clear communication with your doctor is essential

Action Plan

- Ask questions whenever you are unsure
- Avoid relying on incomplete or misleading information
- Follow a balanced, evidence-based approach
- Stay consistent with monitoring and treatment
- Work closely with your doctor

Looking Ahead

Even after answering these questions, some common misconceptions still remain.

In the next chapter, we will address these myths and misunderstandings, helping you separate fact from fiction and make more confident decisions about your health.

Chapter 19: Common Myths and Misconceptions

What People Often Get Wrong and What You Should Know Instead

Even after all the information we have discussed, many patients still carry certain beliefs about cholesterol.

These beliefs often come from friends, social media, advertisements, or partial information. Some sound convincing, but they may not be entirely accurate.

Clearing these misconceptions is important, because **wrong beliefs can lead to wrong decisions**.

Let us look at some of the most common ones.

---

1. "Cholesterol Is Always Harmful"

This is one of the most widespread misunderstandings.

Cholesterol is not harmful by itself. It is a natural substance your body needs for normal function.

The problem arises when cholesterol is out of balance, especially when LDL remains elevated over time.

---

2. "If I Eat Healthy, I Cannot Have High Cholesterol"

Diet is important, but it is not the only factor.

Genetics plays a major role.

Some people have high cholesterol despite eating well, while others may not have high levels despite less healthy habits.

That is why testing is important for everyone.

---

3. "I Feel Fine, So I Must Be Fine"

This is a dangerous assumption.

High cholesterol usually does not cause symptoms.

You may feel completely normal while changes are slowly occurring inside your arteries.

Waiting for symptoms can delay treatment.

---

4. "Once I Start Medication, I Will Be Dependent on It"

This concern is very common.

Cholesterol medications are not addictive.

They are often needed long term because the underlying tendency for high cholesterol remains.

Stopping medication without proper guidance may allow levels to rise again.

---

5. "Statins Are Dangerous"

There is a lot of misinformation about statins.

In reality, they are among the most studied medications in medicine.

Most patients tolerate them well, and serious side effects are uncommon.

---

6. "Natural Remedies Are Always Safer"

Many people assume that "natural" means safe and effective.

While lifestyle changes are essential, many supplements have limited scientific support.

Some may even interact with medications.

It is important to use evidence-based approaches.

---

7. "Cholesterol Problems Only Happen in Older Age"

Cholesterol-related changes often begin much earlier.

Even though complications appear later, the process usually starts years before.

That is why early awareness is important.

---

8. "If My Numbers Improve, I Can Stop Treatment"

Improvement is often the result of treatment.

Stopping treatment without proper guidance may lead to a rise in cholesterol again.

Management is usually long term.

---

9. "All Information on the Internet Is Reliable"

Today, information is easily available, but not all of it is accurate.

It is important to rely on trusted sources and professional advice.

---

10. A Balanced Way to Think About It

The goal is not to create doubt, but to create clarity.

When you understand what is correct and what is not, you can make better decisions.

A Simple Thought to Remember

If you remember one idea from this chapter, let it be this:

Do not let myths guide your health decisions. Let clear, reliable information guide you.

Chapter Summary

- Cholesterol is essential; imbalance is the problem
- Diet alone does not determine cholesterol levels
- High cholesterol usually has no symptoms
- Medications are not a sign of dependency
- Statins are generally safe and effective
- Natural remedies should be used with caution
- Cholesterol problems can begin early
- Reliable information is essential

Action Plan

- Question common beliefs and verify them
- Avoid making decisions based on myths
- Seek reliable medical advice
- Stay informed through credible sources
- Focus on evidence-based care

Looking Ahead

You have now reached the final stage of this journey.

In the next section, we will bring everything together and focus on one clear goal, living a long, healthy life with your cholesterol under control.

Conclusion

Living Well, Living Long, with Cholesterol Under Control

When you first think about cholesterol, it can feel like a complicated and somewhat intimidating topic.

There are numbers to understand, terms that sound technical, and often conflicting advice from different sources. Many people are left wondering,
"How serious is this, and what should I really do?"

If you have come this far, that uncertainty has already begun to fade.

You now understand what cholesterol is, how it behaves in the body, why it becomes elevated, and how it affects your long-term health. More importantly, you now know what you can do about it.

And that is where the real value lies.

---

1. Cholesterol Is Not Something to Fear

Let me begin with a simple but important thought:

Cholesterol is not something to fear. It is something to understand and manage.

When ignored, it can quietly lead to serious problems over time. But when recognized early and handled properly, it becomes a manageable part of your health.

You are no longer guessing. You have clarity.

---

2. Small Steps Lead to Meaningful Change

It is easy to think that improving health requires big, dramatic changes.

In reality, the most meaningful improvements come from small, steady steps taken consistently.

- choosing better foods most of the time
- staying physically active
- maintaining a healthy routine
- taking medication when needed
- following up regularly

Each of these may seem simple, but together they create a powerful effect over time.

---

3. Prevention Is One of Your Greatest Advantages

One of the greatest strengths of modern medicine is prevention.

You do not have to wait for symptoms to appear. You do not have to wait for a serious event.

By managing your cholesterol today, you are reducing your risk of heart attack, stroke, and other complications in the future.

You are making an investment in your long-term health.

4. Stay Connected to Your Care

Cholesterol management is not a one-time decision.

It is a continuous process that involves:

- regular monitoring
- occasional adjustments
- ongoing communication with your doctor

Think of this as a long-term partnership focused on your well-being.

5. Balance, Not Perfection

Life is not perfect, and your routine does not have to be either.

There will be days when you do not follow your plan exactly. That is normal.

What matters is your overall direction, not occasional deviations.

A balanced and sustainable approach will always be more effective than striving for perfection.

6. You Have More Control Than You Think

Perhaps the most reassuring message is this:

You have a great deal of control over your health.

Through understanding, awareness, and consistent action, you can influence your cholesterol and reduce your risk in a meaningful way.

This is not just about managing a lab value.

It is about living with energy, confidence, and peace of mind.

Final Summary

- Cholesterol can be effectively managed
- Early awareness and action make a significant difference
- Lifestyle and medications work together
- Consistency is more important than perfection
- Long-term care and follow-up are essential
- You have the ability to take control of your health

Your Final Action Plan

- Stay aware of your cholesterol levels
- Maintain healthy daily habits
- Follow your treatment plan consistently
- Keep regular follow-up appointments
- Address concerns early
- Stay motivated and focused on long-term health

A Final Thought

Over the years, I have seen many patients take control of their cholesterol and improve their health in a steady and meaningful way.

They did not do anything extraordinary.

They simply stayed consistent, stayed informed, and stayed committed.

You can do the same.

This book was written to guide you, reassure you, and help you move forward with confidence.

Your journey toward better health does not end here.

In many ways, it begins here.

Appendix 1. A Simple Cholesterol-Friendly Food Guide

What to Eat More Often and What to Limit

Many patients feel overwhelmed when it comes to diet. There is too much advice and too many restrictions.

Let me simplify this.

You do not need a complicated diet. You need **better choices, made consistently**.

Foods to Include More Often

Fruits and Vegetables
Aim for variety and color.

- Apples, berries, oranges
- Spinach, broccoli, carrots

Whole Grains
These provide fiber and help lower LDL.

- Oats
- Brown rice
- Whole wheat bread

Healthy Fats
These support better cholesterol balance.

- Olive oil

- Almonds, walnuts
- Seeds

Lean Proteins
Choose lighter options.

- Fish, especially fatty fish
- Skinless chicken
- Beans and lentils

Foods to Limit

Saturated Fats

- Red meat
- Butter
- Full-fat dairy

Processed and Fried Foods

- Fast food
- Packaged snacks
- Deep-fried items

Sugary Foods and Drinks

- Soft drinks
- Desserts
- Refined snacks

A Simple Plate Method

- Half your plate: vegetables
- One quarter: whole grains
- One quarter: lean protein
- Small amount: healthy fats

Key Takeaway

You do not need perfection.
You need **consistency and balance over time**.

Appendix 2. A Practical Daily and Weekly Routine

Turning Knowledge into Daily Habits

Many people know what to do, but struggle with how to apply it.

Here is a simple structure you can adapt.

A Sample Day

Morning

- Light breakfast with whole grains and fruit
- Short walk or light activity

Afternoon

- Balanced lunch
- Avoid prolonged sitting

Evening

- Walk or light exercise
- Balanced dinner

Night

- Relaxation
- Aim for consistent sleep

A Sample Week

- Physical activity at least 5 days
- Mix walking and light strength exercises
- Plan meals when possible
- Allow flexibility without guilt

Key Takeaway

A simple routine followed regularly is more powerful than a perfect plan followed occasionally.

Appendix 3. How to Read Your Lipid Report

Understanding Your Numbers Without Confusion

Your cholesterol report is one of your most useful health tools.

Key Components

LDL
Main number to focus on. Lower is better.

HDL
Protective cholesterol. Higher is helpful.

Triglycerides
Reflect diet and metabolism.

How to Interpret

- Do not panic over a single number
- Look at trends over time
- Consider your overall risk

Questions to Ask

- What is my target LDL?
- What is my overall risk?

- Do I need treatment?
- When should I repeat testing?

Key Takeaway

Your report is not just numbers.
It is a guide to your health.

Appendix 4. Questions to Ask Your Doctor

Making Your Visit More Useful and Productive

Many patients leave the clinic with unanswered questions.

This simple list can help.

Before Starting Treatment

- What is my overall risk?
- What should my LDL target be?
- Can I try lifestyle changes first?

If Medication Is Recommended

- Why do I need this medication?
- What benefits should I expect?
- What side effects should I watch for?

During Follow-Up

- Are my numbers improving?
- Do I need any changes in treatment?
- How often should I follow up?

Key Takeaway

Good questions lead to better care.

Appendix 5. Your Personal Cholesterol Tracker

A Simple Way to Stay on Track

Tracking your progress helps you stay motivated and informed.

What to Record

- Date of test
- LDL
- HDL
- Triglycerides
- Weight
- Notes (diet, activity, medication changes)

Why It Helps

- You can see trends clearly
- It improves communication with your doctor
- It keeps you engaged in your own care

Key Takeaway

What gets tracked gets improved.

Final Note

You do not need to remember everything in this book at once.

Come back to these appendixes whenever you need guidance.

They are designed to support you in real life, not just while reading.

Thank You and

Please Review the Book

Thank you for taking the time to read this book. I sincerely hope it has helped you understand your health a little more clearly and has given you practical, everyday steps you can follow with confidence. If you found this book helpful, **I would truly appreciate it if you could leave a brief and honest review.** Even a few lines sharing your experience can make a meaningful difference. Your feedback helps other readers find reliable, trustworthy health information and supports them in making better decisions for themselves and their families.

Warm regards,
Dr Prabhat Das

Continue your Healthcare Journey

Good health is a journey, not a single step. It is not achieved in one day or with one book. That is why I created the **"Better Health with Dr Das"** series, with each book addressing a different common condition. If you would like easy, practical guidance on other everyday health concerns, you may wish to explore the rest of books in this series.

Books in this series:

- A Doctor's Easy Guide to Understanding & Managing **OBESITY**.
- A Doctor's Easy Guide to Understanding & Managing **HIGH BLOOD PRESSURE**.
- Doctor, What **DIET** Is Best for Me?
- Doctor, Why Can't I **Lose Weight?**
(a Doctor's Guide to safe & Sustainable Weight Loss)
- A Doctor's Easy Guide to **GLP-1 for Obesity**
- A Doctor's Guide to Living Well With **DIABETES**
- A Doctor's Guide to Understanding & Managing **HIGH CHOLESTEROL**
- A Doctor's Guide to Understanding & **Managing THYROID DISEASES**

www.ingramcontent.com/pod-product-compliance
Lightning Source LLC
LaVergne TN
LVHW020854300926
849194LV00002B/12
* 9 7 8 1 9 7 1 6 7 2 1 8 2 *